# Diabetes Knockout!

# DIABETES KNOCKOUT!

## Michael Anthony Hall

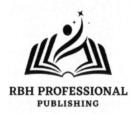

**RBH PROFESSIONAL**
PUBLISHING

RBH Professional Publishing

Southfield, Michigan 48075

Diabetes Knockout!

.

Published by RBH Professional Publishing, A division of

RBH Professional Development Institute
2000 Town Center Drive, Suite 1900
Southfield, Michigan 48075
(866) 600-6322
www.rbhprofessionalpublishing.com

Book Cover Illustrator
Juan P. Bennett

Library of Congress Cataloging-in-Publication Data

Library of Congress Control Number:  2023920785

ISBN: 979-8-9893303-1-7

eISBN: 979-8-9893303-0-0

# Dedication

*This book is dedicated to my grandmother, my mother, my son and all our ancestors who have had to deal with diabetes. This book is dedicated to those who died and suffered medical complications up to and including death, and more frequently having body parts chopped off, for the lack of knowledge. If the phrase "you are what you eat" is true, meaning it is important to eat good food in order to be healthy and fit, then so is the reverse, poor or bad food can make you unhealthy and unfit. I also dedicate this book to my family and friends who have molded me to be who I am. I hope you will enjoy my witty sense of humor while dealing with such a serious topic.*

*My first book, The Hamster Wheel was my Magnum Opus. I guided my readers on a journey to financial freedom. I explained in detail how to hit the stop button on the hamster wheel and leap off into green pastures. It is a great book if I say so myself. I thought that was my greatest work until my 11-year-old son was diagnosed with Type 2 diabetes.*

*I am calling this book my transformative Magnum Opus! My purpose for the information that I share regarding my diabetic journey is to be able to help others transform to a medicine free lifestyle. If you are experiencing Type 2 diabetic issues, this book is dedicated to you as well. I believe it is clear, concise and invokes a plan of attack. Hit me up and let me know what you think.*

## PAY IT FORWARD

*Type 2 diabetes is at epidemic levels all over the world. We need to get this information out fast! Purchase this book for someone who may not be able to afford the book. Simply purchase the book under pay it forward and someone can receive the book for free. You can also share the website which is totally free. Together we can reach everywhere on the globe.*

## SHOUT OUTS!

*Endocrinologists all over the world! I have been hard on you guys; however, we would be lost without you!*

*Barbara O'Neill, I found your info regarding decoding diabetes to be informational, and indicative of a person who really cares!*

*Angry Pharmacist, what can I say, Keep fighting the fight! Dr. Krista!*

*Reversing Diabetes Type 2 Support Group, You guys are da bomb! Keep educating and supporting! Can not say enough about the group and moderators!*

*Mindful Diabetes, dude looked at one video and stayed up all night looking at all the videos. You clearly understand the importance of educating people as to what different foods do to your blood! Kudos to you, my friend.*

*My personal nurse Ruth B, thank you for all of your help and support and yes, I do lol*

*To my big brother, thank you for holding the line while I swing for the fence, luv u*

*Dr. D Abboud (the vegan butcher), thank you for being all about my health. I hope your other patients are inspired. I will speak about reversing Type 2 diabetes wherever you need me. Just throw up the bat signal.*

*Lastly a special shout out / dedication to my seed, she is more like me than any of the boys. As impressive as she is it does not compare to the love I have for my daughter. I Love you, Mimi.*

*My family, there would be no me without them. I love y'all.*

# Contents

# Introduction

Type 2 diabetes is affecting people all over the world! Each year cases are rising. We must stop and take a stand. Diabetes has been plaguing my family, generation after generation. You will find that diabetes is disproportionately affecting certain people. I truly believe this disease is one of the easiest diseases to manage and reverse. How do you touch the globe, how do you save the world? You impact Type 2 diabetes by sharing information and making the information accessible to the entire world.

You cannot make people give a crap, this is true. I **can** share the information to bring about change. You can lead a horse to water, but you cannot make him drink. However, eventually if he does not drink that will be one thirsty horse, and he will be looking for water. The water to reverse your Type 2 diabetes is right here, take a sip, I assure you that it is nice and refreshing! MDOT

Applied Knowledge is Power

El conocimiento aplicado es poder

应用知识就是力量

La connaissance appliquée, c'est le pouvoir

المعرفة التطبيقية هي القوة

Angewandtes Wissen ist Macht

Прикладные знания – это сила

Pengetahuan terapan adalah kekuatan

Kiến thức ứng dụng là sức mạnh

Make no mistake, we beat this disease by spreading accurate information. I believe 3 in 4 adults with diabetes live in low- and middle-income communities. Diabetes and insulin resistance are more prevalent with poor and disenfranchised people. If you learn something from my book, please share it with the world. Go to www.diabetesknockout.com to follow my journey and understand how to reverse Type 2 diabetes. The information on my website is free of charge! We need to get the information out especially to the poor and disenfranchised who may not be able to purchase a book.

**G.O.M.A.D. = GO MAKE A DIFFERENCE**

This book is not meant to give you medical advice. I am simply sharing my journey. The first step in knocking out Type 2 diabetes is to meet with an endocrinologist!

# Round 1

**EVERYONE HAS A PLAN UNTIL DIABETES PUNCHES YOU IN THE FACE.**

My son was an overweight child. My wife nurtured him with food. The two of them are thick as thieves. I'm sure if she knew that the excessive food, sedentary lifestyle, and poor food choices would trigger his diabetic gene, she would have done things differently. There is a lack of education about diabetes that must be bridged.

Years ago, we looked at diabetes as an old person's disease. My son was diagnosed with Type 2 diabetes at 11 years old. Immediately as a parent you go into panic mode. You blame yourself and are ashamed to tell anyone about your plight. My son cried in my arms and said, "why me" and at that time, I didn't have an answer and even if I did, it would not have consoled my 11-year-old son.

**FAST FORWARD 15 YEARS.**

I was at work and a coworker asked if I wanted something

from the store. I requested cranberry juice. When I drank the cranberry juice, I immediately had to pee. I thought it was odd, however, I had no other symptoms, so I shrugged it off. Within the same week rinse and repeat, she asked I requested, drank the cranberry juice, and had to instantly pee. Oh snap! I did not run to the doctor; I did not go see an endocrinologist. I immediately changed how and what I ate and drank. I hated water! I am not fond of it now; however, I drink it consistently. I changed my drink of choice from juice to water. I went all in! All water. Months passed and I had no issues, so I thought. A year later I changed my eating habits. Small changes, more meat, and vegetables and salads.

**DEUCE'S SONG.**

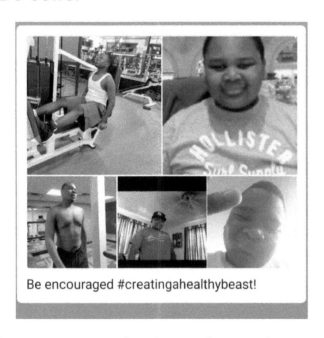

Be encouraged #creatingahealthybeast!

I call my son Deuce. When he was diagnosed, I immediately

immersed myself in the world of diabetes, I researched everything and everywhere. We were going to beat this and get him a reversal or call me Suzie! As of 2023, when it comes to Deuce, people are still calling me Suzie. I guess that is better than Karen.

I learned that through diet and exercise Type 2 diabetes could be reversed, however, there were not a lot of documented reversals. I purchased a treadmill and designed a high intensity interval training program for him. His mother, or shall I call her thief number 1 because he is thief number 2, remember they are thick as thieves, started monitoring his eating habits better. The rest of this part of the story is like child labor. I literally chained him to the treadmill, kicking and screaming. He had to do a mile and a half a day, and if it was not done by the time I got home, which often was late at night, I woke him up and made him run!

## MY THEORY

I researched and found that most diabetics were deficient in mitochondria. My plan was to change his diet and increase his exercise then throw in resistance training to build or create more mitochondria and boom! get his reversal. I never thought it would be so hard. The mental and psychological toll that it takes can seem insurmountable. I never wanted him on the drugs because to me the drugs just masked the problem.

I remember the day the endocrinology nurse explained to him, that if he thought he was going to overeat or eat poor choices to just take a little more insulin. I was livid and did not agree! In my opinion, diet and exercise would be enough. How could the medical community condone drugs to mask the problem.

Sadly, I now understand that most people WILL NOT exercise and eat right consistently to control their blood sugar without medicine. Medical professionals are aware of this, so they are really good at explaining the medicine part, let's just say they put their emphases on controlling diabetes with drugs.

My son lost all the weight, he played on his high school basketball team. Deuce started dating the girls who used to call him fat, he was feeling invincible. Deuce would not take his meds like he was supposed to. He stopped exercising. This is the part of the book where you are saying, I am reading this book to find out information about reversing Type 2 diabetes and it doesn't sound like this kid reversed anything! This is true; however, the story is far from over. Just sit tight and in the end, you will be satisfied (ok that didn't mean go to the back of the book sheeesh! No patience!)

Anyway, this is typical behavior of teen diabetics. They go through grief stages and a lot of emotional baggage that they hate. Imagine if you're the kid that must see the nurse daily to take your medication, that blows! You are different than everyone else. Your friends can eat all the bad things when you all go to the store after school, and you are not supposed to! Freak that, you are eating that Snickers bar and not telling a soul, but your numbers are going to snitch on you!

OK, back to me. I changed my eating habits, every so often I had a bit of frequent urination. When it occurred, I made sure

I would get some exercise in, drink more water, and continue to eat right. In my mind I knew I had diabetic complications but what did I do? I denied it. I knew at some point I had to visit a doctor and have blood work done. In my mind I would get around to it.

Fast forward at least a year later I noticed I was urinating longer than usual, I'm thinking prostate issues, then I had to urinate frequently. Diabetes had not crossed my mind, to me the signs were not clear diabetic issue signs. Well don't you know it got worse, I went and got a checkup. My A1c was 13! They prescribed metformin 1000 mg. WTF, the diabetic bug was confirmed!

At this point I must explain to you that I almost died when I was a wee child from strep throat and scarlet fever. I was about five. I do not have many memories of my childhood, however, the image of me being held down by my brother in the hospital bed so they could put more IVs in my arms is still rather vivid. I recall the veins collapsing and the doctor explaining that they were going to have to stick me in my foot! OH, F@#K NO BATMAN! If you have not figured it out yet, I hate getting stuck. I recall telling people that I will eat lettuce and water every day before I get stuck every day! Well to test your blood sugar YOU HAVE TO STICK YOURSELF!!!

I took my metformin religiously and all my symptoms vanished, I was good, so I thought. I ate right, drank water, and had kind of stopped exercising so much, but no symptoms, I was ok until I wasn't. A diabetic knows when the symptoms start flaring up.

Back to Deuce, he looked good and really did not feel symptoms. We tried everything. We made him look at pictures of amputees due to diabetes. In his mind he could play competitive basketball, he looked and felt invincible. He asked me to put this sentence in my book. Young people just because you *feel* good doesn't mean you *are* good. There were times when Deuce had nigricans on his neck from an insulin imbalance. He has had some neuropathy with one of his feet. None of this was a wakeup call for Deuce. He is better now taking insulin and knowing how to treat his condition, however, he has not mastered his condition. He has still allowed his condition to master him.

# Round 2

## FOR BLACK PEOPLE ONLY

This section, like those images of old racist water fountains is for "Colored Only."

Just as the title of this chapter says, if you are not "colored" just move on to the next section of the book. I don't mean to offend you in any way, but if you are not colored this message is NOT for you. I will give you a moment to process this and move on. (I am playing the jeopardy tune in my head right now)

Okay, it is just us in here right now. How ya'll doing? Life is a bitch, isn't it? How do you feel about seeing the first black (or half black) president? It was cool huh? My 95 year old mother got a chance to see it!

## ALRIGHT LET'S TALK ABOUT THIS DIABETES THING.

My guess: If you are reading this you know someone, friends, family members, and/or enemies who have diabetes. Some of you know people who have had limbs amputated and unfortunately have died from diabetic complications. Supposedly, Ella Fitzgerald and Thomas Edison are a few who fell victim to this paralyzing disease.

Diabetes disproportionately effects African Americans. Why?

*Conspiracy Brother: Well Michael, that is a no brainer. The white man created diabetes to kill us off. This is similar to the likes of the Tuskegee Syphilis Experiment and COVID! Anybody can write a book sheesh!*

Conspiracy Brother, I don't think that your line of thinking is totally accurate especially when it comes to diabetes, allow me if you will.

If you look at who diabetes affects the most, you will see that it disproportionately affects poor people (Briggs et al., 2021). I present to you that diabetes is NOT racist. I repeat diabetes is NOT racist. Diabetes is prevalent in situations predicated by poor food availability, poor food choices, and a lack of knowledge concerning healthy living coupled with a sedentary lifestyle.

Allow me to take you back to my sweltering hot summer Detroit days as an adolescent. We played outside in the sweltering heat for hours only to run inside and grab a glass of refreshing Kool-Aid! Like in many ethnic families, the Kool-Aid recipe was passed down carefully from generation to generation.

This formula's concoction consisted of getting the correct fusion of the little Kool-Aid packages (food coloring), a ton of freaking sugar, and a little water. In our household, the Kool-

Aid was primarily made by my big brother. Owee that Kool-Aid sho was good! And now years later, we have learned what exorbitant amounts of refined sugar can do to your body. We had no idea just like most things we ate and drank. We lacked the knowledge to make better food choices.

I'm sure there are similar stories resonating throughout many poor and middle-class households. Further, the link to unhealthy diets and diet restrictions dates back years into our history. Let's talk about slavery. Do you think the slaves said, "No massa we don't want that slop tonight. We will take a balanced carbohydrate diet with enough protein and fiber. Add a cool refreshing glass of water. Thank you." Hell no! They didn't have a choice. Hence, unhealthy food choices and patterns began way back then. These unfit dietary regiments have been passed down generationally. Here we are today.

**FAT BABIES**

Okay, I am about to talk about ya'll fat babies and get canceled. There is nothing wrong with a fat baby. I had one. Babies are growing humans and need ample nourishment during those fat baby years. However (here it comes), if you keep overfeeding those babies in conjunction with the lack of monitoring the types of food you are giving them, what do you think is going to happen? You could be setting them up to be fat diabetic toddlers or an insulin resistant child. In order to change the diabetic narrative, there has to be a change in the dietary components to which we expose our children.

Change! Unfortunately, people despise change. Humans do not like change. But the need for change is in high demand.

## JOY'S SONG (YOU CAN LEAD A HORSE TO WATER)

Joy worked with me for years. One day she shared with me that she had been suffering from Type 2 diabetes. I immediately started giving Joy advice and pressuring her to make better food choices. This went on for at least a year and she just would not make the necessary changes to alleviate her diabetic symptoms.

This was excruciating for me because I cared for Joy like a daughter. One day we were conversing, and she recalled a time when she was on her way home waiting for the bus. Without any warning, Joy went blind as she awaited the arrival of her bus/WTF! Yes, she was blind for an entire day due to complications triggered by her diabetes. Did she change her eating habits and exercise after that? Will a fat baby refuse cake?

Joy's experience is close to many of our own. A wise man once said, "if you know better, you do better". Yet, so many of us know what is right for our health, but we continue to do the opposite. Imagine if you warned 1000 smokers that the consumption of one more cigarette would result in immediate death. You can take an educated guess on what would happen. You would have some happy dead smokers!

*Not true, Massa was good to us. They had to give us good food to survive working in the field all day. Michael, you're just stirring this slavery thing up with lies. Hell, anybody can write a book.*

## *UNCLE RUKUS*

The truth is we need to learn how to make informed food choices and the role exercise plays with our bodies. There is a Facebook group I belong to called Reversing Diabetes Type 2 Support Group. The people in this group, especially the moderators, are AWESOME! They preach WOE (Way of Eating). People in that group have reversed their diabetic numbers and some have done it by just changing what and when they eat. I reversed my numbers through diet and exercise. They count carbs and support each member through better food choices! Big ups to yall in the group, they had no idea I was writing a book when I joined.

The work that is being done in this group has been very impactful. So much so, I have created my own derivative of WOE. My distinctive diabetic science is WOE & E: Way Of Eating and Exercise!

Public Service Announcement: Don't think I don't know there are non-colored people in here just cause y'all are sitting back being quiet! I'm not stupid!

*Smart educated brother: So, if you're not stupid how do we fix the generational issues of poor food, poor food choices, and lack of education? You so smart!*

## WE MUST BREAK THE CYCLE!

Well smart educated brother, I propose we treat diabetes like the nation treated COVID, especially in the poor areas. We spread the information. It begins with individuals acknowledging that diabetes is somewhat innate and there is not a specific action that causes its existence. We trigger it through poor food choices and a sedentary lifestyle. We need to tell everyone it is okay to be diabetic and it is one of the easiest diseases to deal with. In the time that we spend being embarrassed and hiding our diabetic condition, we could be rolling up our sleeves and getting to work to put it in remission.

Did you know that diabetes is reversable? I can almost guarantee that a poll of 10 people, will yield results that will determine only a single person realizing that this is a reversable disease. However, of the ten, not one person will be able to identify one who has documented their diabetic reversal. We then have to spread the word that diabetes can be reversed. Applied knowledge is power! Diabetes education should be mandatory in every school, specifically in the poor and disenfranchised areas around the world. Make no mistake I see Diabetes as a global epidemic We need to get more people talking about "Reversing Diabetes."

Exposure on all platforms is necessary to spread the word. We need more celebrities coming out and opening up about diabetes. Well known American actor Anthony Anderson has been beating the drum regarding Type 2 diabetes. He has been going hard! If I could speak with Mr. Anderson, I would thank him for everything he is doing. This is not without reminding him that I remember when he was fat. Lol! Oops. I'm getting canceled again. Allow me to summarize.

Acknowledge that diabetes has genetic qualities; therefore, you have done nothing wrong. There is nothing to be ashamed of. Speak out about reversing your condition! Scream it to the mountaintops. Type 2 Diabetes is reversable! You can reverse your diabetic numbers. Your pancreas has the ability to heal.

We must introduce the information in our schools. Through diet and exercise, you can prevent Type 2 diabetes from triggering. Join groups like Reversing Type 2 Diabetes on Facebook.

Share this book. I will come and speak with schools, churches, and organizations. Please reach out. My info will be somewhere in this book lol.

Remember, Type 2 diabetes can be reversed through diet and exercise!

# Round 3

## EXERCISE!

Did you say exercise? Are we talking about exercise? Yes, Allan, we are talking about exercise!

"Humans are so intelligent they are killing themselves quietly" Mdot

*Here you go again with the BS. I knew I should not have read this book. What tha he!! are you talking about? Anybody can write a book!*

## SKEPTICAL GUY

In many cases your body has been overloaded with sugar for years. We must relieve the pressure of the sugar overload and give the body a chance to heal (correct itself). Get that excess sugar out of your system by any means necessary!

Well skeptical guy, please allow me to elaborate. I live in Philadelphia. I spend a fair amount of time on a pedal bike. When I was reversing my diabetic numbers, I had to work exercise into my schedule. What better way to burn off sugar and increase mitochondria? While I'm pedaling around Philadelphia I would see electric bicycles, electric scooters, and electric skateboards. In short, I see any and everything that allows the person to not exercise and use up sugar and stored fat in their body! In my opinion exercise is needed to maintain your bodily functions just like water! I believe that proper exercise helps every part of your body work properly.

I also believe the body is made to be in motion, whether the body is sick or healthy. I have taken plenty of 3 day getaways to isolate myself so I could eat right and exercise without distractions. You must create good habits to replace the bad habits. Eating right paired with cardio and resistance training is the formula. Sometimes twice daily. Your workouts must be challenging! Make sure you challenge yourself with each workout.

Use every chance to get exercise or activity. Park your car away from the store and walk. Walk or ride a bike. Take the steps instead of the elevator etc. Don't make life easy. Get a jump rope. Do push-ups. And sit ups. Go for a walk each day for 30 minutes.

## LET'S TALK COVID!

*Ooh here we go with the BS! I knew the moment he mentioned Covid this was gonna be some government conspiracy ish! Hell, anybody blah blah blah*

## CONSPIRACY BROTHER COUSIN

If you look up Covid deaths in the United States alone it is in the millions!

Well, I believe that our response to COVID is what killed so many people. The big issue with COVID was the mucus increasing inside the lungs. What was our response? Bring the patients in and lay them in a hospital bed. What did that do? Well, it allowed the mucus to keep increasing. In my opinion, we should have never laid people on their backs. People should have been sitting up and getting steam treatments to loosen up the mucus. If able, patients should have been walking around. They should have been receiving hits on their back to help loosen up the mucus. It is my belief the human body is made to be in motion. When you take away that motion, it creates problems for your body. I believe not getting enough physical activity can lead to heart disease, obesity, high blood pressure, high cholesterol, and more.

## WHAT DOES EXERCISE DO TO YOUR SUGAR?

Exercise allows the body to use glucose. Your sugar can be high in the 300s, but exercise can bring that number down. Hold on Karen. Yes, I am aware if you are in the 300s you should go to the ER. Trust me, I have lived this life. High sugar counts effect people differently. I have personally had blood sugars over 300. As a result, I exercised and then witnessed it dropping over time. This is not the ideal way. Rather, it is a risky solution. It would have been nice to have had some metformin or insulin, however, neither of them was at my disposal at the time. After an exercise session your sugar will spike, (avoid carbs or sugar after exercise) and it should come down. Exercise burns off sugar.

I burned off my overall sugar through exercise while simultaneously cutting carbs and sugars. I exercise regularly as maintenance. Hence, I am in Vegas as I am writing this. This morning I had a low carb breakfast, water, and coffee with sugar substitute. I know. This is my guilty pleasure. Normally I use monk fruit. I am sitting by the pool at 1:00 in the afternoon and my Continuous Glucose Monitoring device (CGM) says 90. Later tonight, I might go back to the gym after I eat and lose more money. Lol.

I believe a regular exercise routine is essential to your body's health. Do you remember when you were little and you played Double Dutch, rode your bike, played football, basketball, and baseball? I still remember my legendary leap when I played kick ball. People did not know I had hops like that! When we were young, no one had to tell us to exercise!

Let's look at today. How many kids are outside playing (cricket sounds)? A lot of them are sitting around playing video games, barely moving, and becoming a sitting target for diabetes. We need to develop a video game called triggering diabetes and use that to educate them on the disease! Trust me, it would be a whole bunch of triggered diabetics *in* the game while *playing* the game!

In My Samuel Jackson Voice: "Motherf@#ker! Get the f@#k up and get yo butt out there exercising now! Move your motherf@#king butt." Use this as motivation every time you stick yourself. Think about this every time you are urgently urinating or when you have fruity breath with the metallic taste in your mouth. Or even when you watch your loved ones struggle with the symptoms.

*Wow, sound familiar? I know bro. Been there, done that! Writing a book about it. Lol, Did I mention that Type 2 diabetes can be reversed through diet and exercise?*

- 1) Purge the excess sugar out of your body by exercising. I do a mile and a half on a treadmill or ride my pedal bike. I also do resistance training with weights.

- 2) Stop putting sugar and carbohydrates in your system as much as you can. I went cold turkey. Every diet professional will say there is a better way to reduce your carbs. Blah… blah…blah. I went cold turkey. I needed the excess sugar out of my system, like yesterday!

- 3) Always consult an endocrinologist. This is not simply medical advice; this is how it should be done. I primarily eat meat, vegetables, and salad.

- 4) Get a Continuous Glucose Monitoring device (CGM). The information that is provided is immeasurable on your journey to reverse your condition.

- 5) Be a maniac about your diet. Exercise ( watch

your sugar and carb intake) the first three months and in about three more months, your numbers should be in range, maybe sooner. You will no longer need medicine and you will have reversed your condition. As long as you control what you eat and never overload your body again, your numbers will no longer be in the diabetic range.

## THE GYM

As I have explained, I understand the importance of exercise. As a result of my Type 2 diabetes, I have become a gym rat!

Previously I explained that I believe the human is so intelligent that we are killing ourselves slowly. You wake up in the morning and say I need to go to the gym to exercise. From the moment that you open your eyes you are already lying to yourself. Your brain has begun the f@#kery!

*Michael, what do you mean?*

For most people, exercise is not fun for your brain. Being that exercise is just the opposite of fun to your brain, your brain will figure out ways to avoid it at all cost! "I need to go to the gym to exercise" is a lie from the pit of he!! (say that phrase like an old Black woman) To exercise you simply need to get up and get down on the floor and do push-ups or sit ups or other isometric exercises.

You do not need the gym, but your brain says "If I can trick him/her into thinking they **need** to go to the gym, I have more time to find excuses for them **NOT** to get there. If you work out regularly you can recall a time when you had a piss poor effort. I pulled up in front of the gym before and never made it in. When I run on a treadmill, after a minute my brain begins to tell me to stop. My brain says the following:

1. *After 1 minute*: Stop this is enough

2. This is good enough. You do this like every day!

3. Just do a mile today. It will be okay.

4. Your foot is hurting. Don't run today.

5. Your shoestring is becoming untied. *Stop* and fix it.

I can go on and on. My brain is very intelligent and knows how to manipulate my own thinking. I power through and ignore it 99% of the time. YOU MUST MASTER YOUR BRAIN. Put it this way, if exercise was sex, it would be a whole lot of healthy people walking around smiling. Your brain would be figuring out ways for you to exercise continuously. This same master manipulation can apply to exercise. Make it your will.

Muhammed Ali was once asked about his road work. He danced around the question examining how far he ran daily. He is rumored to have said "I just run as far as I can until I cannot run anymore, and then I run back!" Those who know "the greatest" is well aware of his keen sense of humor. Yet, if you remember those grueling matches where you thought he would not last due to his body being physically beaten, you now know why he answered the bell time after time!

## MASTER YOUR BRAIN!

I suggest you immerse yourself in the gym world. Find a workout partner. A workout partner can motivate you and keep you honest. Some people need that shame from blowing off exercise. Thereby disappointing your workout partner. You need to be a part of a gym community of people that are trying to live healthier. You need to join groups and converse with like-minded people. It can motivate you! Surround yourself with positive like-minded people.

Presently, I am keeping my numbers low and allowing my pancreas to heal itself. This was, of course, before yesterday. Ugh! Did I mention, I am in Vegas? Well, what goes on in Vegas, stays in Vegas! For the most part, I have been adhering to my diet until yesterday! I ate at Carbone and had margaritas on the strip. My numbers were all over the place. I just knew that I had shot my sugar up to 280. Fortunately, *I did not and they stayed in range.* More importantly, they would gradually go up after meals or drinks and come right back down within the hour. WTF! I was pleasantly surprised. Praise GOD! Sometimes you should be allowed to live life! When I get back to Philly, I will be back on my strict life of healthy diet and exercise.

A true total reversal or putting Type 2 diabetes in remission requires a sugar test to be administered. You need to see, after you have given your pancreas enough time to heal, if it handles sugar and carbohydrates properly. Essentially, getting your body off of the medicine is a win in and of itself; it is considered a reversal. Getting a documented reversal and putting Type 2 diabetes in remission, in my opinion, is the ultimate win. I'm sure that will be my second book. Lol

## FOR FAT PEOPLE ONLY!

Yes, you read it right. This section is for fat people only! Yea, I'm about to get cancelled so I will wait for the nonfat people to leave. (Cue Jeopardy theme song again)

OK, let me start by saying I am 5 feet nothing and weighed 190 lbs. I was fat! The insurance company scale said I was obese. I say this to let you know that all of the insults and information you are about to undergo in this chapter is with genuine love and compassion. For some of y'all, somebody should have told you this **ish** a long time ago.

This is for the ladies who get dressed and ask their dude "Does my butt look big?" His response should have been, 'I love you but he!! yea. Not only your butt, look at them great-grandma arms. They look like you cook chitterlings every day. And them mutherf@#kin kancles. They look big as ish!"

Of course, this never happens. The now high divorce rate would be unimaginable. Let me qualify how I look at Fat People. If you are fat and have zero to no health issues coupled with no predisposition to diabetes, you are fine with me. This section is not for yo big attractive self. After all, big gurls are in!

If you are bigger than a Buick and have health conditions due to weight, this chapter is for you! This same logic applies to the fellas that played football in their glory days, gained all that weight trying to be big, and now you're stuck huge and unhealthy as f@#k. What if Godzilla was stomping around?

You couldn't run a city block! Godzilla stomping dat butt. Did I get my point across? Ok, let's talk about eating and food.

At some point, especially in America, partly because of capitalism, our food portion sizes became distorted. How much does a human need to eat? I do not know the technical answer but in my opinion, it is a whole lot less than Americans eat now. In Philly, the Philly cheesesteak is a staple of the city. There are places that one cheese steak could feed the entire Jamaican bobsled team!

Further, I have sat down with friends, colleagues, and acquaintances and listened to them brag about the amounts they eat. I see this all the time. People consistently brag about the portion size of food establishments. What do you think most of these people look like? What happens when you eat too much? I believe it causes excess fat if you do not exercise properly. I believe it can lead to metabolic issues such as insulin resistance and if you are predisposed to diabetes, you will trigger it. A result of eating too much is being five foot nothing with the shape of a meatball. Well, maybe that is an exaggeration. But you know what I'm getting at.

Currently, I am at the Cosmopolitan Hotel. I just ate at the buffet. In front of me was a group of four people. They have enough food on their table to feed the poorest third world country. Of course, they just happen to be minorities and I can see their ancestors in their faces. I would guess there is a genetic predisposition to diabetes in at least one of their families. Whatever happened to only eat until you are full.

Somewhere in American History that idea went right out of the window.

*Extremely Large Person: Okay, but let's get back to the exercise information. I am extremely obese. I auditioned for my 600-pound life and they said I would have to lose 600 pounds to make the 600 pounds for the show. How the he!! am I going to exercise? I knew this book was some BS, he!! ………*

Well extremely large and in charge person, you can exercise anywhere. You can use your arms to get your heart rate up to a sustained pace for exercise to begin working on your body. Are you familiar with the Loch Ness Monster? I know the truth about the Loch Ness Monster. Water displaces the volume of water equal to our volume which exerts a buoyant force on our bodies in an upward motion. You feel lighter and move easier in water.

Water removes the pressure from your joints. A water workout is 100% recommended. Let's just suppose there was a giant mammal swimming in the lake. You would not think this mammal would be swimming due to its massive size. Let's say this mammal had to breathe while it swims under water by surfacing its trunk. *Hmmm sound familiar??* If an elephant can swim in a lake, you need to get your big a$$ in some water and do water workouts!

# Round 4

## WHAT WE EAT

The American hamburger must be the most popular food in America. An average cheeseburger and fries has about 102 grams of carbohydrates. Carbohydrates turn into sugar to fuel your body. Too much prolonged sugar that (for whatever reasons) is not being processed properly is not good for your body. This can lead to health conditions including triggering those with the genetic disposition for Type 2 diabetes.

So what should we be eating? I am not a nutritionist. I would suggest you eat more vegetables and salads to give your body more of the minerals it needs if you have not been doing so. I would suggest that you watch your carbohydrates like a cat waiting patiently to catch a mouse. There are good carbs and bad carbs. Please do your research. This book is guiding you toward that research. I already told you what I did to reverse my Type 2 diabetes. Always seek professional advice.

I advocate for the consumption of the Mediterranean Diet. This diet is comprised of mostly vegetables and whole grains, beans, lentils and nuts. In the beginning of my reversal, I cut out everything! I find that on a low carb diet hunger seems to linger around more often, especially at the beginning of the diet. As I settle into the diet, the urge dwindles. I am not a foodie though. I do not love food. I am aware how some people have addictive relationships with food. Your brain knows the taste of the sugar that you have been feeding it most of your life. Nothing can really substitute that refined white sugar. It seems as if sugar is more addictive than most drugs. Your brain will try any means necessary to trick you into giving it sugar. I eat an Atkins bar when I have those cravings.

## "EAT EVERYTHING ON YO PLATE"

Poor families typically do not have a lot of food to waste. Therefore, parents urge children to follow the "eat everything on your plate" rule. Parents will validate the rule with "We don't have food to waste." What if at that moment you lack a robust appetite, yet, your mom piles food on your plate. This shared philosophy is promoting overeating. Do you think that this habit may follow you throughout life? You may begin to believe that overeating is acceptable. We must change this narrative. It is acceptable to take a doggy bag home from the restaurant. Besides, every foodie will tell you that the food tastes better on the second day. Portion control people!

## MAKE NO MISTAKE THIS IS A TOTAL LIFE CHANGE FOREVER!

I have mentioned earlier that we knock out diabetes through

the sharing of information. Information is key to reversing this disease. Before I write about medicine, allow me to share some sources which are worth the price of this book alone. For those people dealing with Type 2 diabetes, this information is priceless!

- 1) Barbara O'Neill can be somewhat controversial on certain subjects; however, I believe that her Decoding Diabetes video on YouTube is spot on!

- 2) The angry pharmacist on Tik Tok is worth watching. She speaks about diabetes and healthcare amongst other interesting issues. Follow "Angry Pharmacist" on Tik Tok.

- 3) "Mindful Diabetes" on Facebook tests foods and shows viewers the impact that these foods have on blood sugar. Knowledge of how foods effect your blood sugar is immeasurable!

Check all three of these out and let me know what you think!

The Facebook Group Reversing Diabetes Type 2 Support Group includes individuals who have successfully reversed their diabetes due to altering their food choices alone! Please check them out and inform them that you heard about them in a book written by Mdot!

I got into a debate with someone in the healthcare business. Yes, I said business!

Do you have any idea how much revenue is acquired

through treating Type 2 diabetes with medicine in the United States? Me either. But it is a big business.

If there is a health care professional who purchases my book and does not learn anything, I will refund their purchase and give them 100 dollars! I believe the treatment of diabetes in the United States alone is a billion-dollar industry. It suddenly makes a lot of sense to keep yo a$$ on medicine, doesn't it?

## MEDICINE

My sugar was stuck up in the 400s! I tried my exercise trick, and it was not working. I was nervous. I went to urgent care, and they did not have insulin. I had no medical insurance. I made a phone call and received fast acting and long-acting insulin. I looked up the dosages and stuck myself. I thought insulin was the magic pill. My sugar would come down some and go up some. I took larger doses of insulin thinking that my sugar would come down and stay down. This all occurred over a 4-day period. I remember taking 16 units.

I eventually got my sugar down and learned that insulin does not remove the sugar from your blood. It lowers it temporarily. This is why you must keep taking it for it to continuously work. Essentially, if you do not do something with the core problem of all that sugar in your blood, you will be trying to control your blood sugar levels with medicine for the rest of your life. In my head there is a place for medicine. **Medicine should be used as a tool to control your levels while you purge your body of sugar through diet and exercise!**

## HYPOGLYCEMIA

Low blood sugar. A regular fasting sugar supposedly should be from 70 to 99. This may change depending on the source, however, we will go with this. I remember the first time my sugar lingered around 100 and then one day it went to 95. I was shocked. You would have thought that I hit the lottery. Then my sugar dipped to under 70. My CGM alarm sounded, and I was shocked. More seriously, I was scared to go to sleep. What if it dipped in my sleep and I died? *Okay, calm down dummy (me).*

I did more research and found out that when your sugar drops low, your body has an almost immediate response and sends sugar into your blood stream. In my case, my body regularly sends around 40 mg into my blood stream. I slept better after it continuously happened. It doesn't happen often, however, think about the fact that I have gone from 400s to having to worry about hypoglycemia! He!! Yea! Most of the articles you read about hypoglycemia will reference diabetics on medicine.

I have been off medicine for months now. I know people who are on medicine and experience blood sugar dips overnight. Yes, it can be scary. Some of the causes can be a malfunctioning CGM device due to you sleeping on it, bumping it, temperature and more. I have experienced the dips after intense exercise at times. People on Keto diets also experience this when glucose in their liver may be low. The other thing is to make sure your CGM is giving you accurate readings. I am using the Libre 2 and 3 for my numbers. I will have official blood work done in about a month in a half. Of course, I will share my results with you on line.

# Round 5 (Knockout)

**NUMBERS**

I have witnessed diabetics whose numbers were so high they could not be taken on a regular glucose meter. Many of the meters at the pharmacy will not display a number if a patient's glucose is too high. Instead, the meter will simply read as "Hi". This is an indication that further expertise is needed to address the glucose levels. In many cases, the hospital is the next route.

If you go to the hospital, they can read the number. I have witnessed people with numbers in the 600s and above. You would think they are the walking dead! Please understand most of them are not blind and have all their limbs. All people are different and unique. I know people who have had numbers in the 300s and complained of blurred vision, headaches, and more symptoms. My sugar in the 300s gives me little to no symptoms.

As it rises, I get all the symptoms with the exception of headaches. When my A1c was 13 the doctor told me I needed to lose weight and take other medicine. He did not even look at my chart. The moment that he saw the A1c he assumed the rest. I weighed 175 pounds at the time. I had lost 15 pounds. I questioned the nurse who upon examining the paperwork apologized for the doctor. Remember, per the insurance underwriting numbers, I was obese.

Numbers are just a guide or a range for you to use to your benefit. I have used the Libre 2 and 3 CGMs. Early on I tried to stick myself and just could not do it. I am going to have official blood work done. I will use those numbers to review and evaluate my condition. I hear people arguing and complaining about the accuracy of CGMs verses blood glucose stick machines. In my opinion, do your research check, and choose one. Be consistent and in the end only go by your official blood work.

## CONCLUSION

I reversed my Type 2 diabetic numbers by diet and exercise.

You can too!

- 1) Purge the excess sugar out of your body by exercising. I do a mile and a half on a treadmill or ride my pedal bike. I also do resistance training with weights.

- 2) Stop putting sugar and carbohydrates in your system as much as you can. I went cold turkey. Every diet professional will say there is a better way to reduce your carbs. Blah… blah…blah. I went cold turkey. I needed the excess sugar out of my system, like yesterday!

- 3) Always consult an endocrinologist. This is not simply medical advice; this is the way to do it. I primarily eat meat, vegetables, and salad.

- 4) Get a Continuous Glucose Monitoring Device (CGM). The information that is provided is immeasurable on your journey to reverse your condition.

- 5) Be maniacal about the first three months and in about three more months, your numbers should be in range. You should no longer need medicine and you will have reversed your condition. If you control what you eat and never overload your body again, your numbers will no longer be in the diabetic range.

YOUR NUMBER ONE GOAL SHOULD BE TO RID YOURSELF OF THE NEED TO TAKE DIABETIC MEDICINE. PERIODT!

**Diabetes Myths**

Myth # 1

Type 2 diabetes skips generations.

Tell my deceased grandmother, my mother, myself and my son that lie! Smh! All of us have it! In my case my current numbers say I'm no longer diabetic as I control it through diet and exercise. I do not eat excessive carbs or refined sugar anymore. I never will again. I take no medicine and my numbers stay in the normal range.

Myth # 2

There are no carbs or sugar in meat and vegetables. Tell that to my CGM as I watch meat and vegetables raise my blood sugar slightly. Yes, meat and vegetables have carbs. They just do not a have lot. Almost everything we eat in the United States either has sugar or carbs. The key is to learn what to eat, when to eat it, and what really was the Loch Ness Monster.

Myth # 3

In your elderly black woman voice: *You done ate all that sugar and done got the diabetes!* read it again… ok you got the joke? I believe that this is a fallacy surrounding diabetes. I believe diabetes is genetically passed down. There is nothing you can do to get diabetes; you are born with it. You can trigger it mostly through poor diet choices and a sedentary lifestyle. Simply put, you can't go and get it if you don't already have it. Sorry mom dukes.

Myth # 4

All fat people have diabetes. *It is 2023 can I use the word fat? Well, I did! Jump in the picket line.* This myth is simply ignorant and untrue. If you watch the TV show "My 600 Pound Life" you will see that all the large and in charge persons were not diabetic. Neither is every sumo wrestler diabetic. There are plenty of skinny diabetic people. What I want to know is, how do those 600-pound people wash their private parts? You know what I'm saying? Just a thought.

Myth # 5

"I don't have insurance, so I cannot get diabetic medicine and glucose machines." There is this thing called the internet that I believe was created by Al Gore. Maybe not. Either way, there are plenty of sites that will hook you up. They even have medical staff that will set you up for an evaluation from a licensed physician. The physician can then write you a script and fill it for whatever you need. I did it!

Myth # 6

It is better to hide the fact that you are diabetic from friends and family. Not true. I get it. I did it. Remember, you have done nothing wrong to get diabetes; it is genetic. There is nothing to be ashamed of. In fact, it is time to roll up your sleeves and get to work. We all need to work together to knock out diabetes. The knockout begins with the sharing of information. Hold your head high. Say "I have diabetes" out loud! You didn't do anything wrong! Say it loud "I HAVE DIABETES!!" SAY IT!! There you go. I am proud of you. Now, let's get to work! (Yes, I really did hear you).

All of you have enjoyed blooper scenes from our favorite movies. The following is stuff my publisher insisted that I leave out of the book, so I left them out lol

## STUFF THAT DID NOT MAKE IT IN THE BOOK.

1. **Conspiracy Brother:** "De Whiteman gave yo ass Diabetes"

2. I wrote, applied knowledge is power in all of these languages and cannot read any of them. Who knows what they really mean? Where did I get this idea? Ugh!

Everyone has a plan until your foot gets cut off!

The rest of the part of this story is like slave labor. I treated my son like Kunta Kinte from the movie "Roots".

If you eat like shit and live a sedentary lifestyle, diabetes is waiting for you around the corner with a smile on its face. He will be your best friend while you go blind and have limbs cut off.

I'm sure this book will get me canceled so if I'm going to get canceled, I'm going to do a great job of it.

This section is for skinny people with diabetes only, Damn, y'all. WTF, eat right and do resistance training! Skinny Bitches...

Follow this plan for weight loss... you Jabba the Hut!

People are walking around right now with a 300 glucose reading and don't even know it. Facts!

They say hide information in a book because some of y'all won't read books.

Follow an ignorant kid home and you're more than likely going to find ignorant parents or an ignorant parent. Follow a fat kid home....

This book is not for everyone! If I do this right, you will be more motivated than ever to DEFEAT DIABETES!

I feel bad for whoever I pay to edit this book!

I read an article in Ebony Magazine written by Jazz Keyes. Kudos to Jazz Keyes!

We look at our a1c numbers like they are credit scores. Lmfao!!!!

In the beginning, the side effects of your diabetic condition will make you lose weight. Use that to your advantage when it happens. Ramp up your diet and exercise. You will be pleased with you results! Take a bad situation and turn it into a good situation.

"Lord please take diabetes from my son. If anyone has to have it give it to me." Shit! We both end up getting it! Who said God does not have a sense of humor?

Mdotyouafunnymutha Shut yo mouth!
Youtube Channel coming soon.  Simply Mdot.

# About the Author

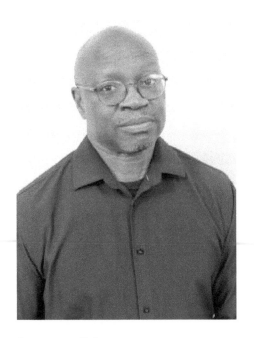

Michael Anthony Hall has an Associate Degree in Biblical Studies from the Center of Urban Theology located in Philadelphia, Pennsylvania. He is proud to say he is from Detroit Michigan. His first book entitled The Hamster Wheel guided his readers to financial independence. His son being diagnosed with type two diabetes at 11 years old set him on a mission to understand and help people rid themselves of the lifelong medicine used to control diabetes and live a healthier lifestyle. Readers will enjoy his uncanny wit and humorous observations while dealing with the worldwide epidemic of Type 2 Diabetes. Should you embark on this journey it will be life changing.

To learn more please visit

www.diabetesknockout.com

To schedule Micheal Anthony Hall

for speaking engagements, or other interests, please contact:

Delorahtyler@firstmediagroup.net

248-354-8705

Milton Keynes UK
Ingram Content Group UK Ltd.
UKHW020931231123
433129UK00016B/833